101
To Know

C.N.A.

Compiled by Neil Shulman, M.D. & Zoe Haugo

Illustrated by Michael Swaim

ISBN: 1-892157-04-7

Copyright Neil Barnett Shulman, 2002

All rights reserved. Rx Humor, 2272 Vistamont Dr., Decatur, GA 30033

Published by RX HUMOR
2272 Vistamont Dr., Decatur, GA 30033

Copyright, 2002 by Neil Shulman
Illustrations by Michael Swaim

All rights reserved. No part of this book may be reproduced in any form or by any means without prior written permission of the Publisher, except brief quotations used in connection with reviews written specifically for inclusion in a magazine or newspaper.

Printed in USA
Library of Congress Number: 2002096343
ISBN: 1-892157-04-7

OTHER BOOKS BY NEIL SHULMAN

Fiction
The Backyard Tribe
Doc Hollywood
Finally...I'm a Doctor
Life Before Sex
Second Wind
What? Dead...Again?

Non-Fiction
Your Body, Your Health
Your Body's Red Light Warning Signals
Better Health Care for Less
The Black Man's Guide to Good Health
High Blood Pressure
Let's Play Doctor
Understanding Growth Hormone

Children's Books
The Germ Patrol
Under the Backyard Sky
What's in a Doctor's Bag?

Videos
*The Real Doc Hollywood Unlocks
    the Mysteries of Hollywood*
What's In a Doctor's Bag?

**See www.dochollywood.com to order, or contact Rx Humor at 2272
Vistamont Dr., Decatur, GA 30033, Telephone # (404) 321-0126**

DEDICATION

*To the Certified Nursing Assistants of the world,
who are a glowing light of compassion, and make a huge contribution
to the health of Americans.*

ACKNOWLEDGMENTS

*Thanks to Senior Vice President of Clinical Services at Mariner Health Care
Jennifer Kulla, and to the following wonderful C.N.A. Council
who contributed to this book:
Sonia Aronson, Florida Bonner, Ginette Boursiquot, Joyce Brown,
Mae Bush, Olivia Clark, Arthur Coard, Ludivina Cravotta, Edy Del Aquila,
Chris Dvorak, Teresa Edwards, Barbara Fox, Angelita Garay, Anita Gonzalez,
James Huffstutler, Gloria Jarrett, Marion Johnson, JoAnn Jordan, Shelly Lauch,
Lorine Legrand, Kim Mack, Katie Martin, Martha Nevarez, Melves Paige,
Janie Quintanilla, Phyllis Simmons, Fili Sonora and Florence Wofford*

1. You begin using a protein supplement
     in your cereal.

2. You have an activities calendar posted at home for your children.

3. You wear your gait belt to the grocery store.

4. The phone rings at 3:15 on your day off and you know exactly who it is before answering.

5. Everyone in your family has an emergency buzzer beside their bed.

6. You open salt and pepper packets
for your husband at restaurants.

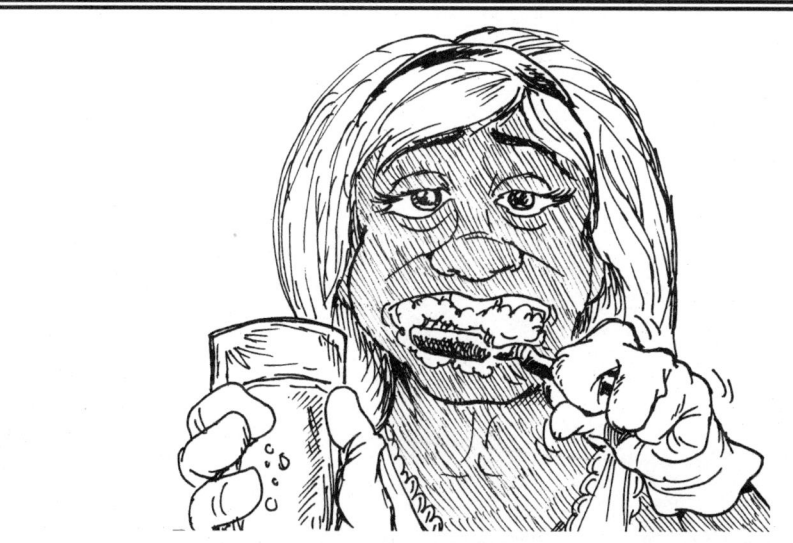

7. You put on gloves before doing anything.

8. The door bell rings and you ask your husband to answer the call light.

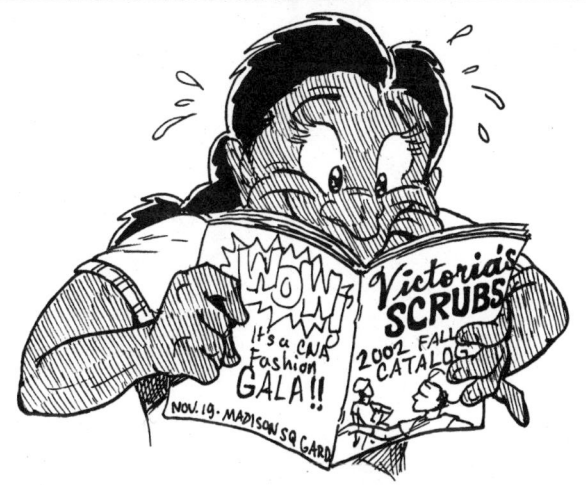

9. Your idea of going on a shopping spree is to look through a scrub uniform catalogue.

10. You use urine specimen cups as knick-knack holders.

11. You want to hug the administrator every time survey day is making her anxious.

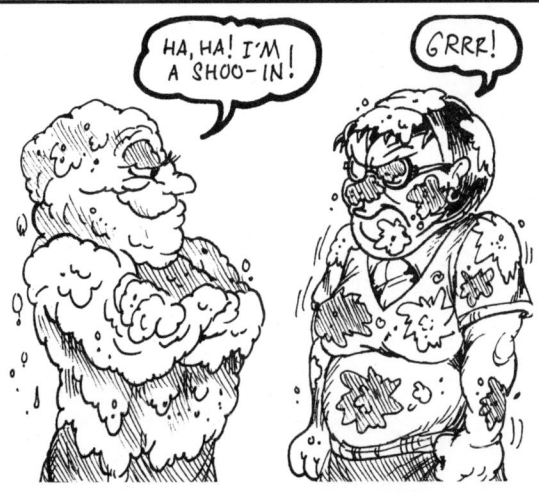

12. You have contests to see who is wearing the most food by the end of lunchtime.

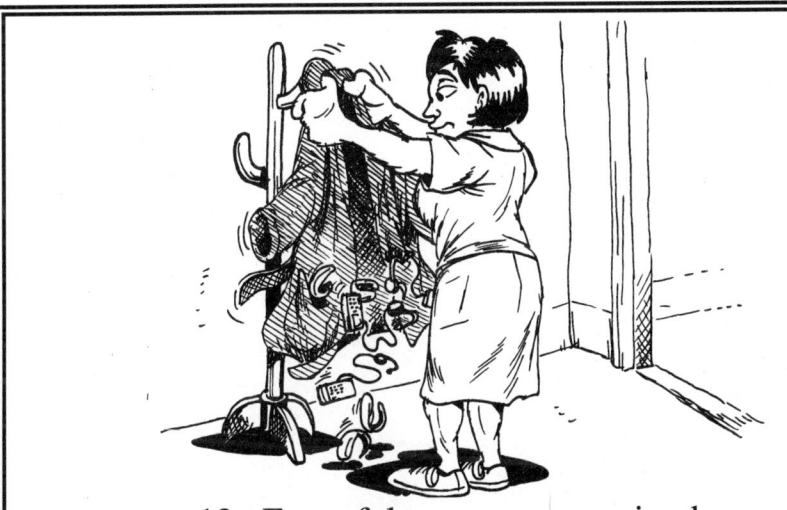

13. Forgetfulness means coming home with a pocket full of hearing aids.

14. You measure your own B.M. as small, medium, or large.

15. You try to lock the brakes on your shopping cart at the grocery store.

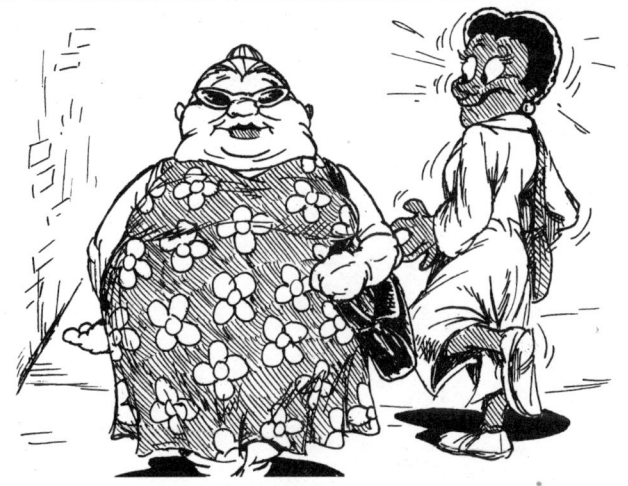

16. You size people up in public on how difficult they would be to transfer.

17. You identify your own urine by color, odor, and amount.

18. You sit in a restaurant and play "Guess the Diet Card" on the other people there.

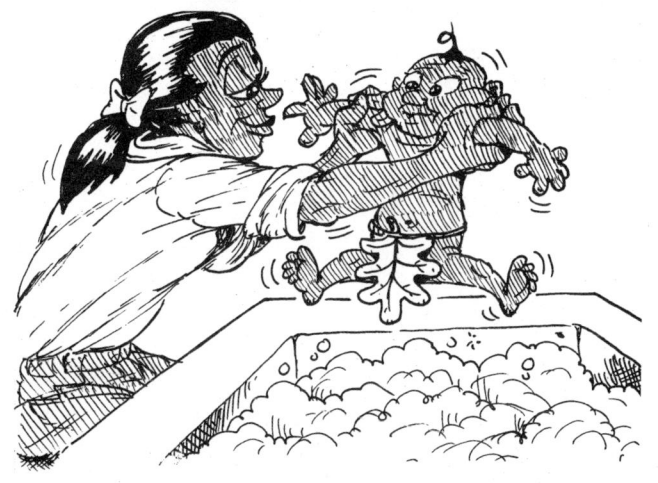

19. You cover your kid's private parts when you give them a bath.

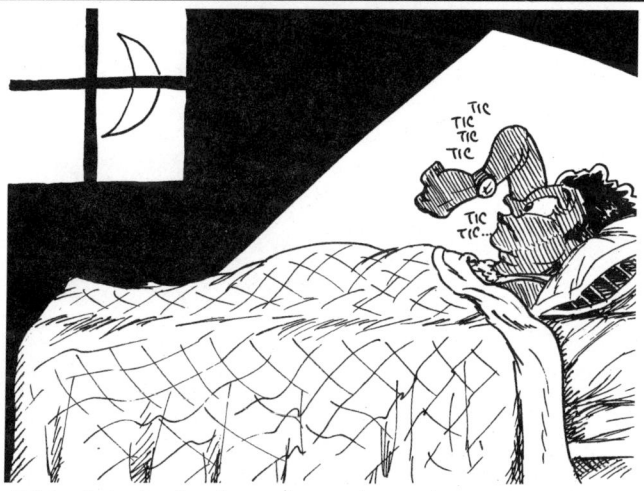

20. You lay in bed and see how long you can stay in one position without moving.

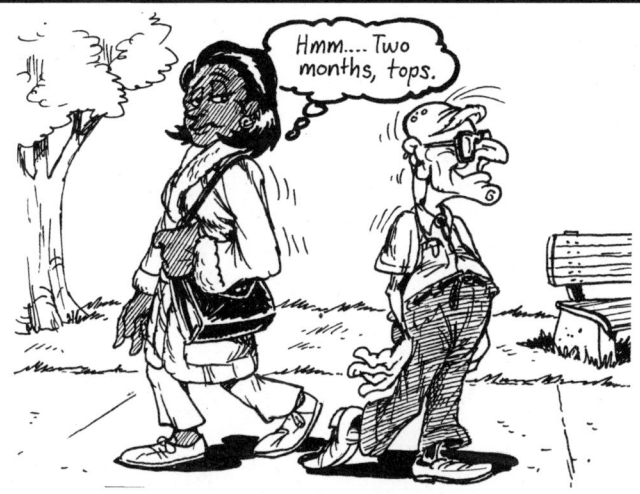

21. You guess at how long before people you see in public end up in nursing homes.

22. You spontaneously jump out of bed
in the middle of the night to answer a call light.

23. You feel too tired after a long day of wiping other people's behinds to wipe your own bottom.

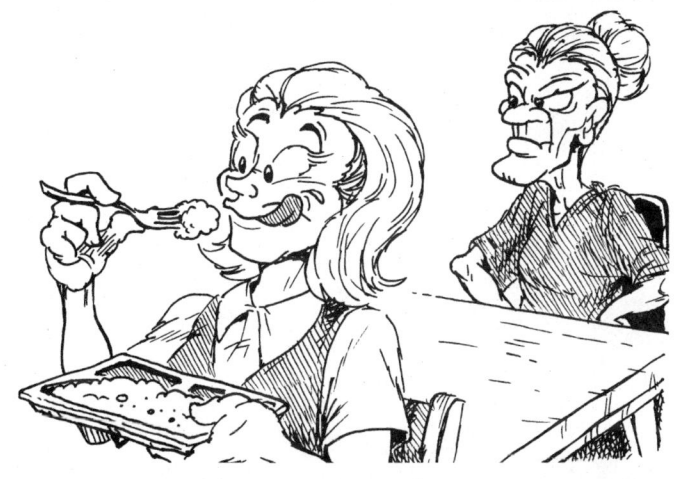

24. You're so hungry that the resident's puree lunch actually smells and looks good to you.

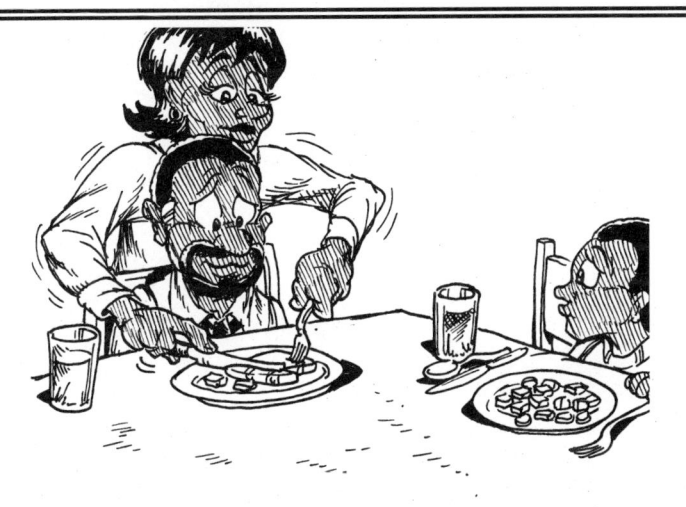

25. You sit down for dinner with your family and start cutting up their food into bite size pieces.

26. You are home alone and knock on the laundry and restroom doors before you enter.

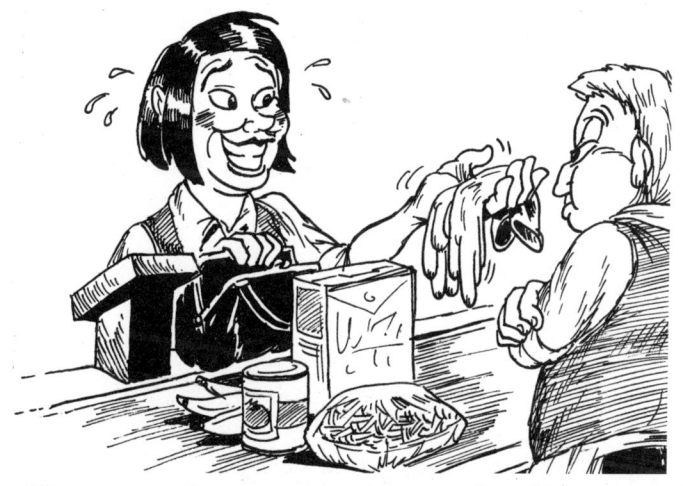

27. You go to the grocery store and pull out a pair of gloves from your purse instead of cash.

28. You have a very big bladder.

29. You make "Care Cards" for your whole family.

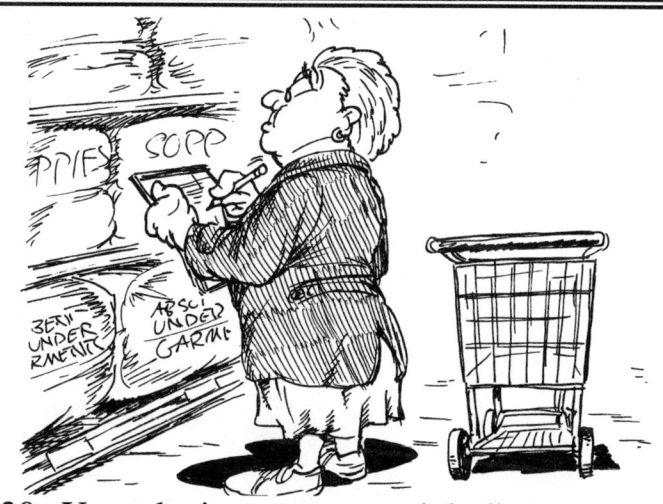

30. You take inventory on adult diapers in the grocery store.

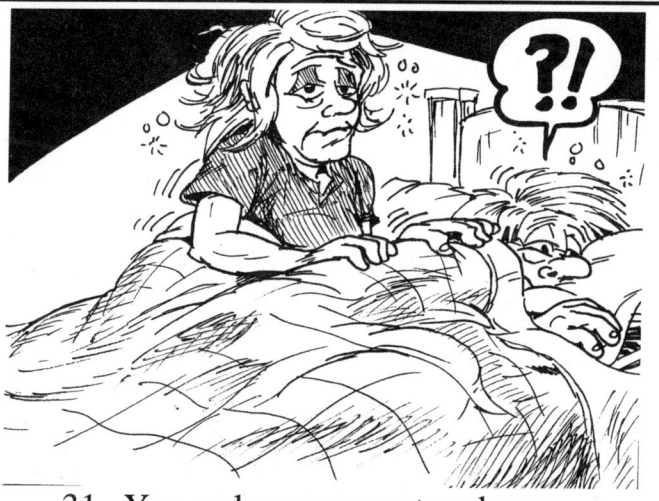

31. You wake up every two hours to turn your spouse.

32. You make your teenagers go to the toilet every 2 hours.

33. You do a "range of motion" on your spouse
in the bedroom.

34. You put clothing protectors on your family.

35. You keep detailed charts of all your interactions with your children.

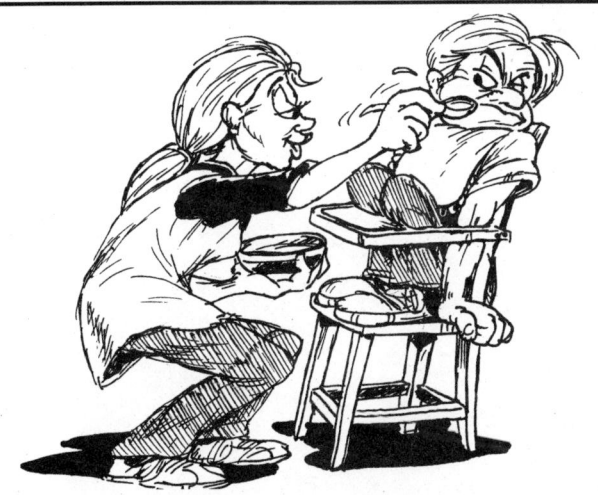

36. You put a bib on your grown children and try to feed them.

37. Your kids complain of a stomachache
and you get a full set of vitals.

38. You have an I. & O. sheet behind your own bathroom door.

39. You scold your kids for playing with their gum and tell them that it's an infection control issue.

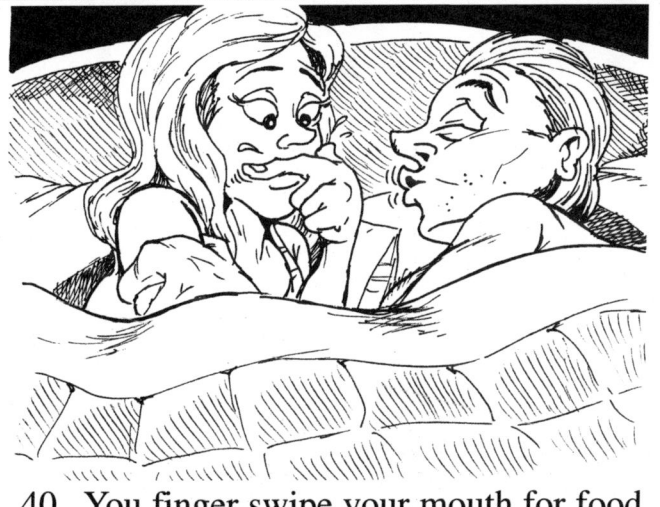

40. You finger swipe your mouth for food prior to a kiss.

41. You buy your child scrubs for school clothes.

42. You have your family on Monday, Wednesday, Friday bath schedules.

43. You chart your kids' input and output every day.

44. You can name three brands of prune juice.

45. Your kids are playing rough and you call it R.O.M.

46. You have your weekend chores on a "flow sheet."

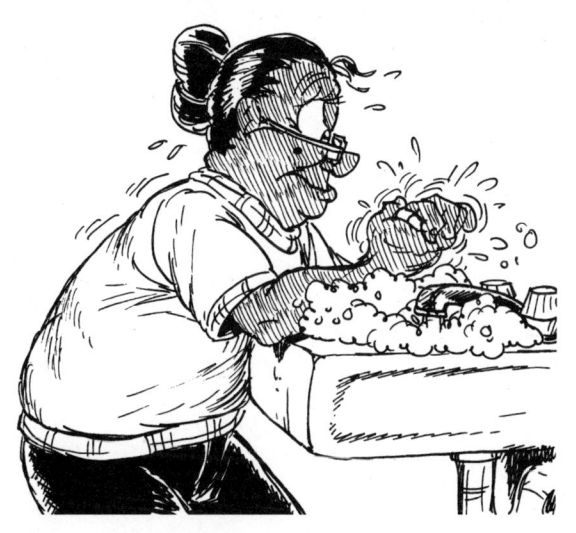

47. You're always washing your hands.

48. Your extended family includes a lot of C.N.A.'s.

49. You regularly check your own behind for breakdown.

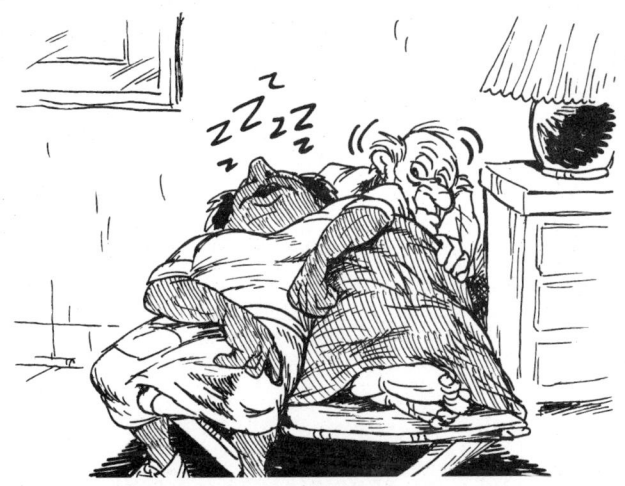

50. You're so tired you ask one of your residents to move over and make room for you on the cot.

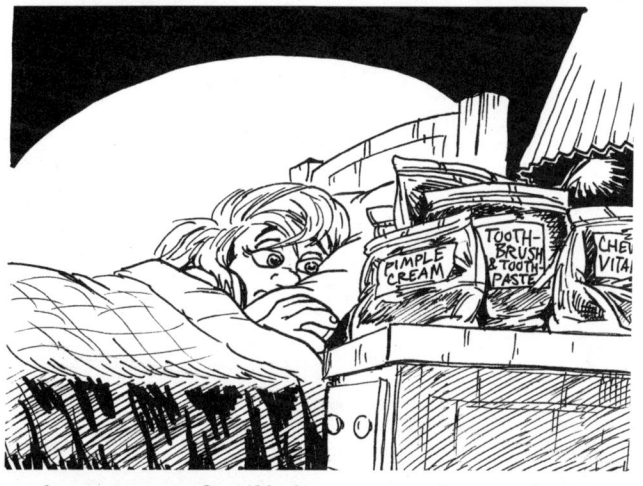

51. You keep your family's personal care items stored in labeled zipper-locked baggies beside the bed.

52. You love to see a nurse smile.

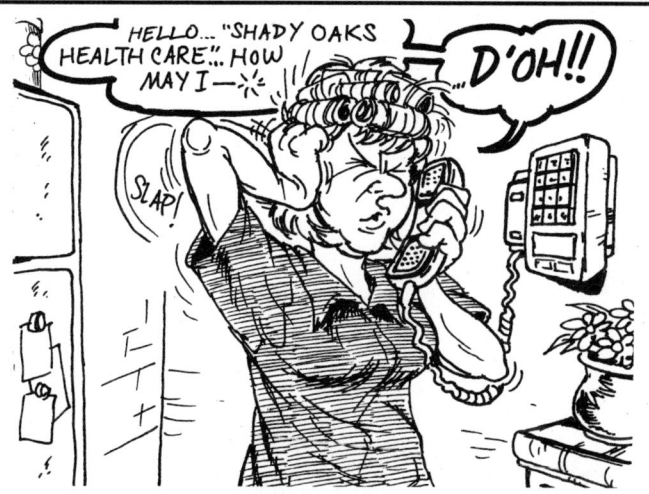

53. You answer the phone at home with the name of your care facility.

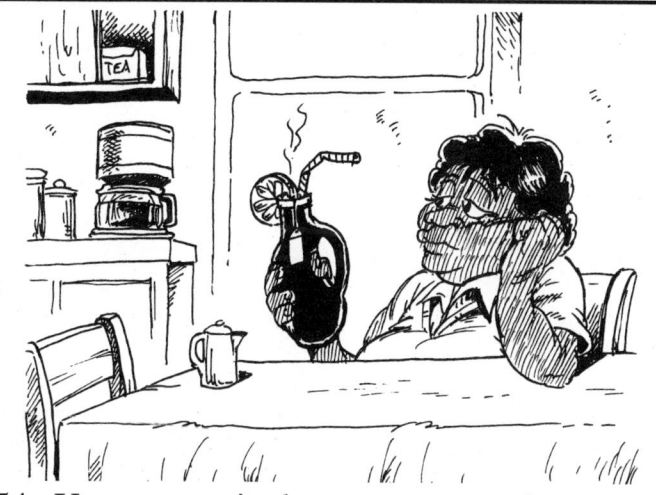

54. You use a urinal as a mug to make sure you're drinking enough water.

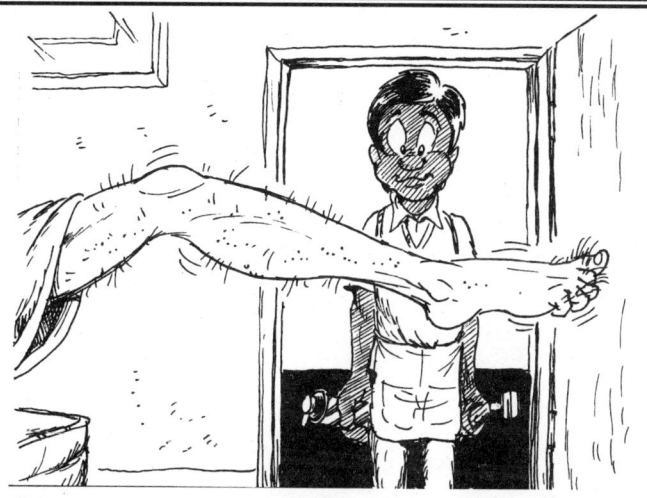

55. You are a master at shaving other people's legs and toes.

56. Your work is to love, kiss, and hold people.

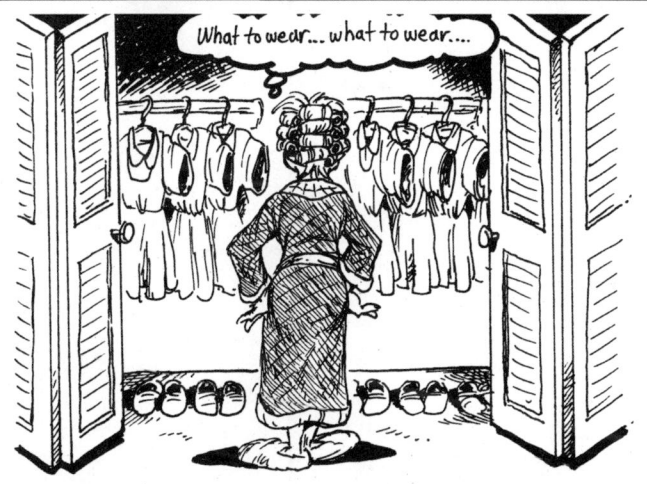

57. You have more uniforms than regular clothes in your closet.

58. You make someone smile every day.

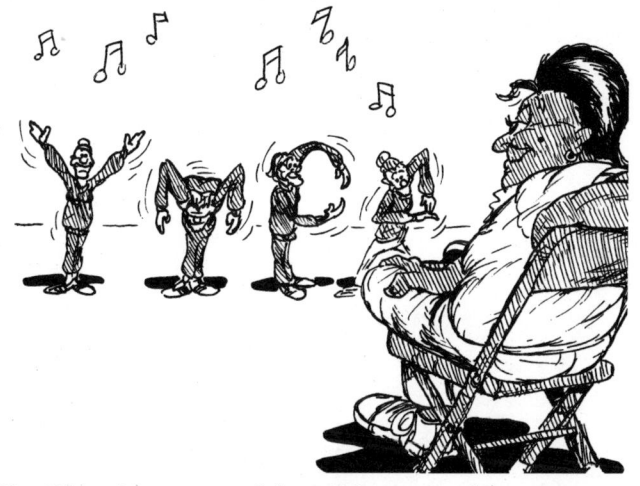

59. You love watching 90 year-old women do the "YMCA."

60. You've got friends who are over 100 years old.

61. You weigh everyone in your family once a week.

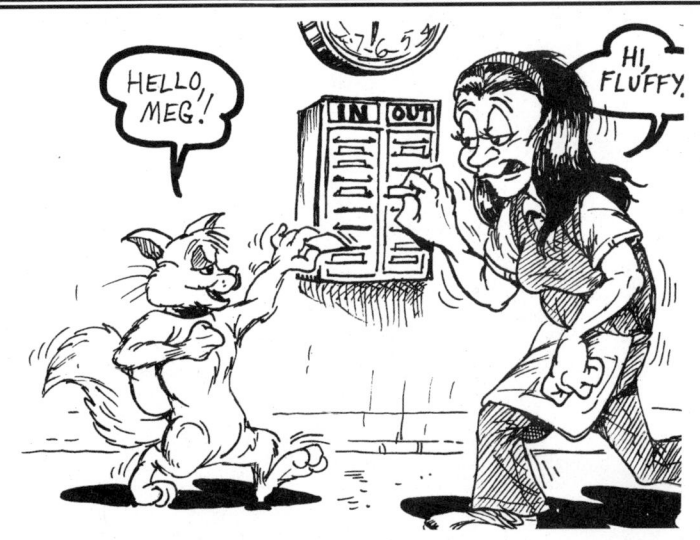

62. Sometimes you get replaced by a nice pet.

63. You label and date left-over food at home.

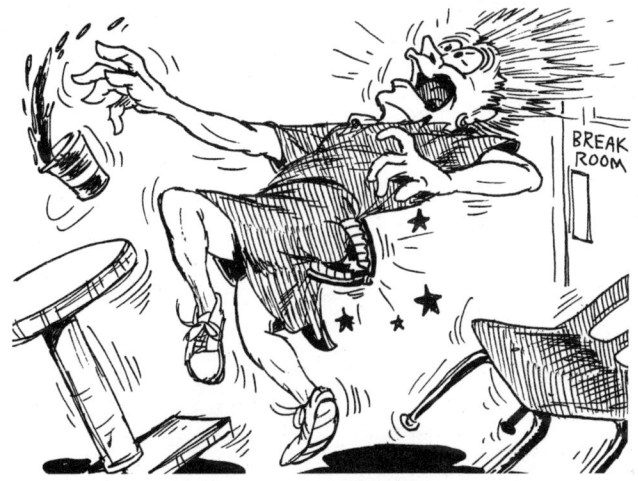

64. One of the unwritten duties in your job description is to help find lost teeth.

65. You play a lot of Bingo.

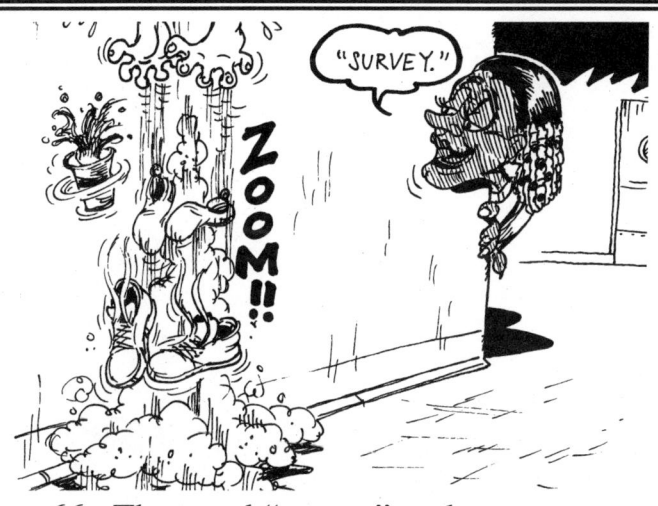

66. The word "survey" makes you jump out of your skin.

67. You have a family of children who are all over 70.

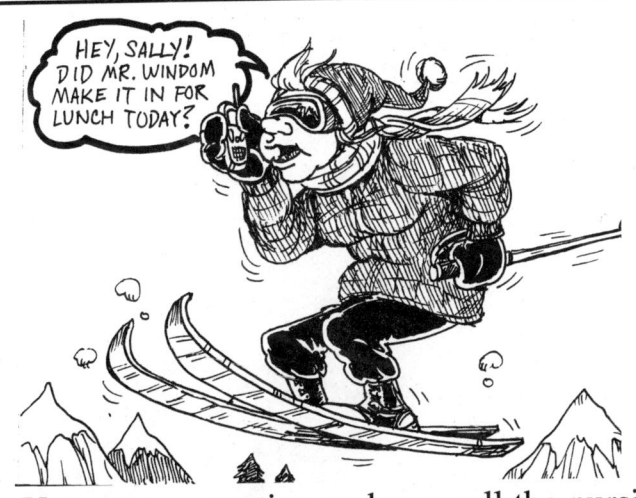

68. You are on vacation and you call the nursing home and ask if your resident ate lunch today.

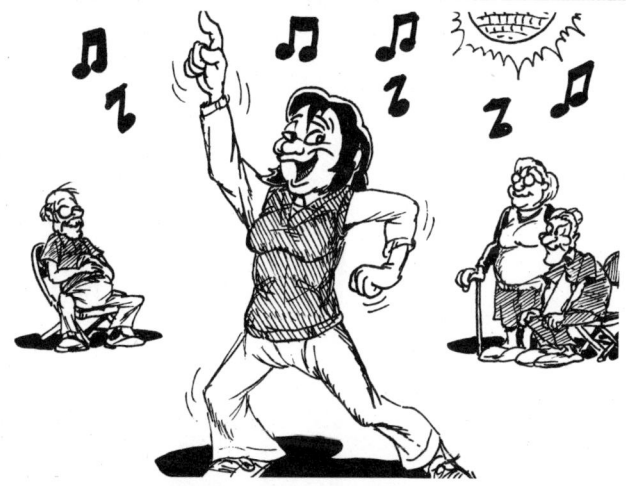

69. You find yourself spontaneously dancing in front of the elderly.

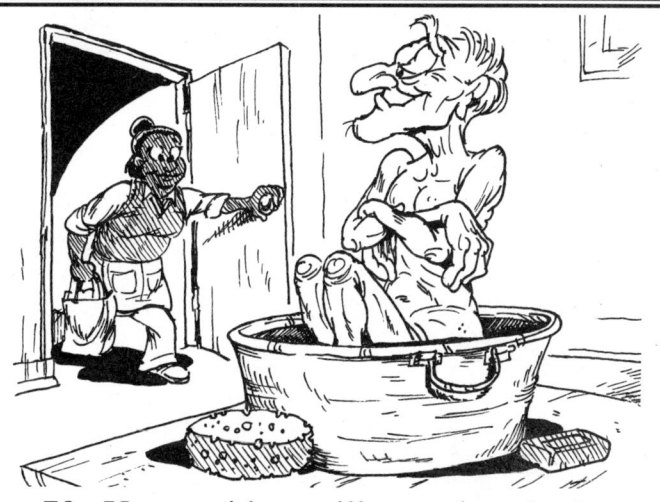

70. Your resident will not take a bath unless you come to work.

71. Every time you take a bath you feel like you're at work.

72. You can't go for 3 days without giving somebody a bath.

73. You ask your husband if he's put on clean shorts every time he gets out of the bath.

74. Your college child needs help on a class brief and you give him/her an adult diaper.

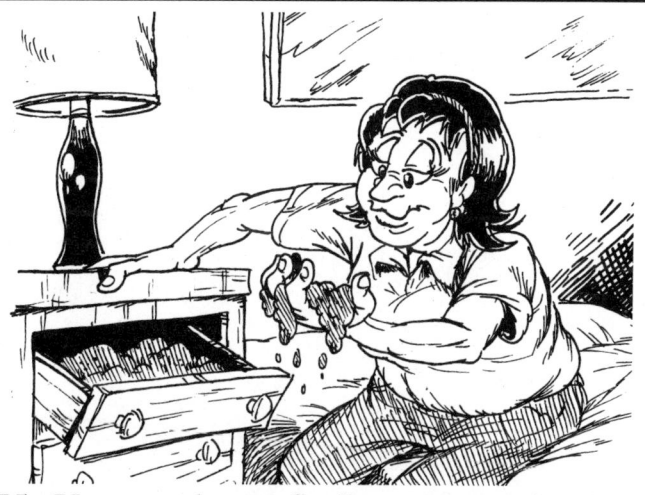

75. You are always finding uneaten food in interesting hiding places.

76. You buy clothes to match the colors of your gait belt.

77. You regularly check your children for their hydration status.

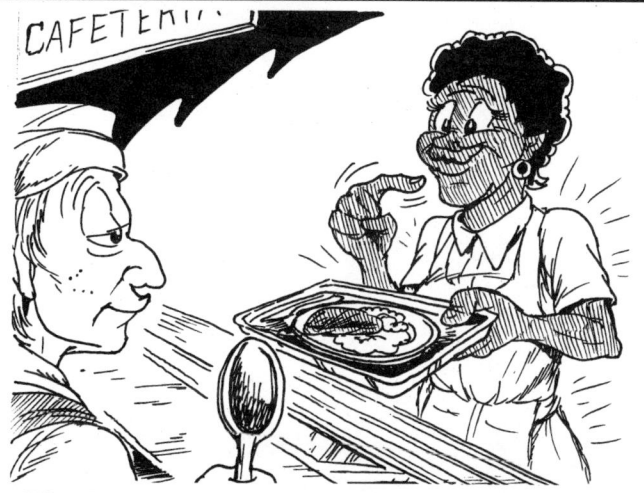

78. You wear your uniform and dine in hospitals so you can get a cafeteria discount.

79. The residents ask you if you ever go home.

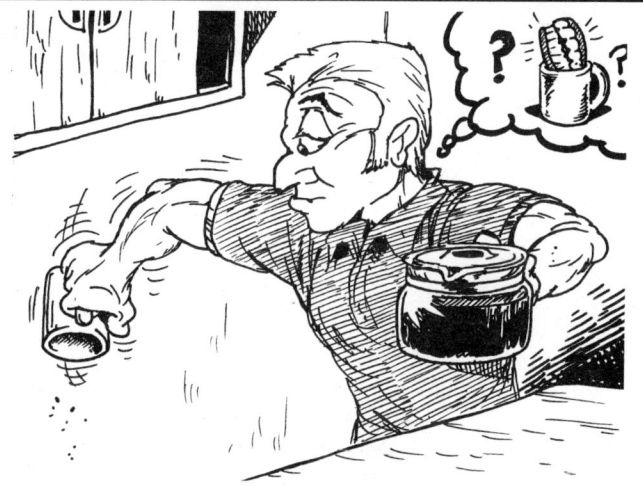

80. You start to see every cup on every shelf as a denture cup.

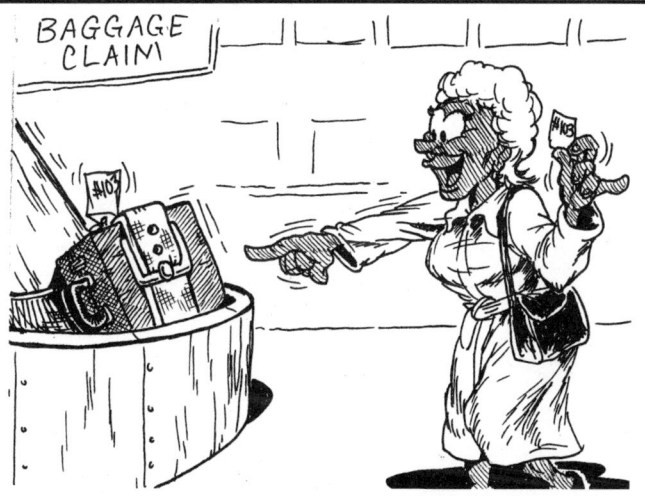

81. You use your gait belt to identify your luggage at the airport.

82. You sign checks with C.N.A. after your name.

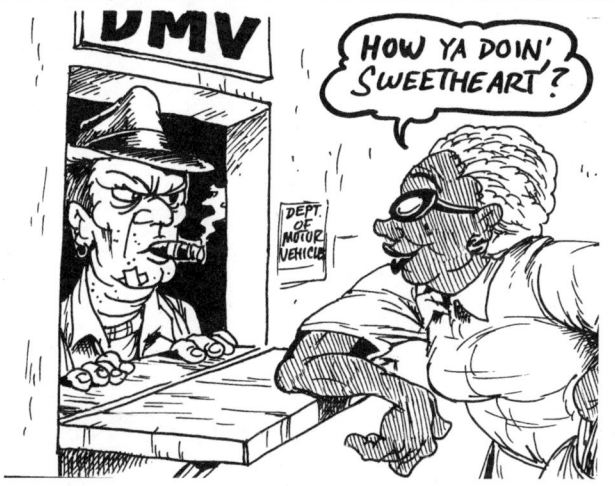

83. You start to call everybody "Honey" or "Sweetheart."

84. When you make a personal visit to the doctor while in uniform, the nurse puts you to work.

85. You clean your white shoes and realize that the brown spots aren't mud.

86. You use your gait belt to help your children walk.

87. Whenever you eat you put a bib on your chest and your lap.

88. You measure the percentage of each food group left over on your family's plates at the end of the meal.

89. You take a "daily shower" 10 times a day.

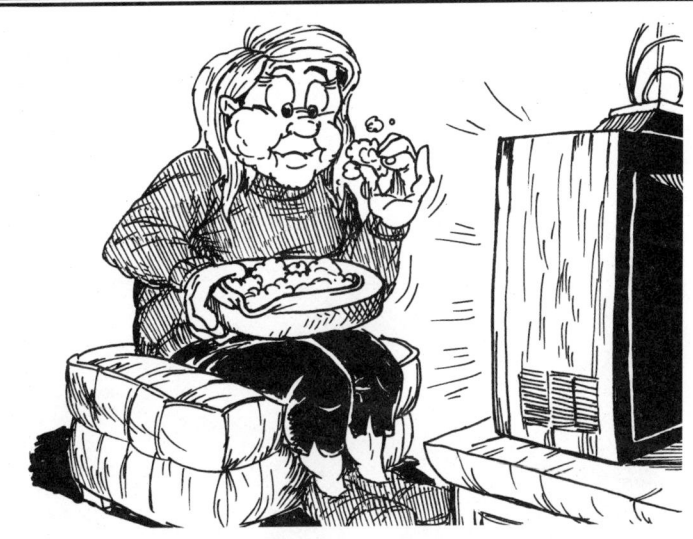

90. You eat popcorn out of a bedpan.

91. You're seeking H.S. care for yourself.

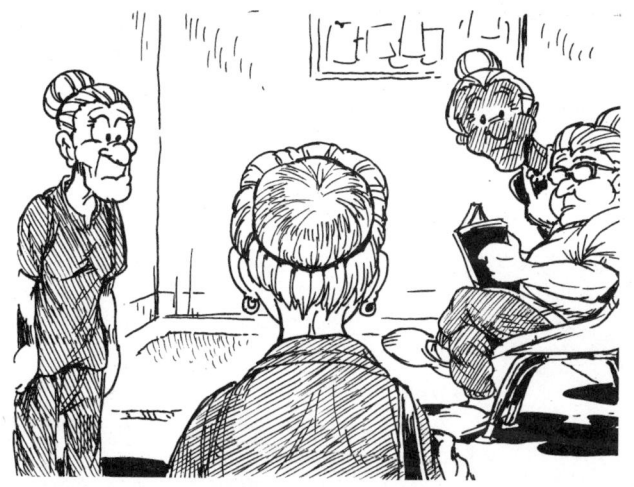

92. Your hairdo begins to look the same as that of all the residents.

93. You begin performing mouth-to-mouth resuscitation when you kiss your mate.

94. You weigh all your children once a week.

95. You make a point of never playing Bingo
on your day off.

96. You are ready and willing to give a back rub on a moment's notice.

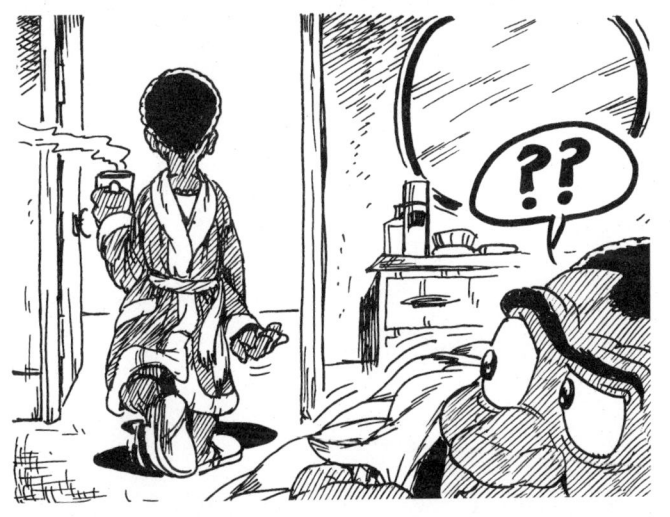

97. You begin to wear your bathrobe backwards.

98. There's nothing worse than emptying your pockets at home and finding a set of dentures.

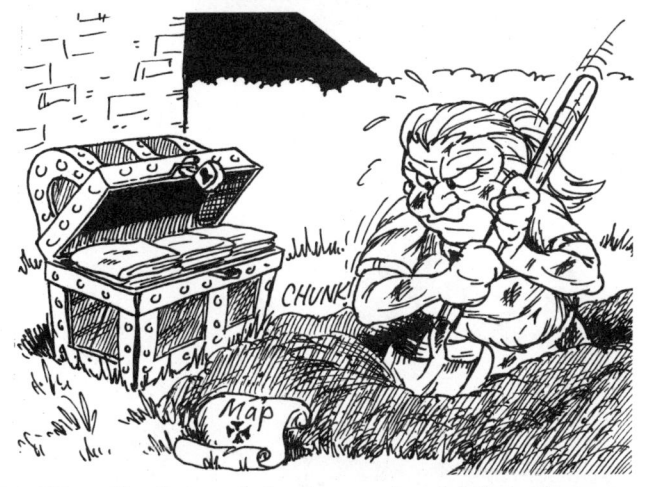

99. You find special places for hiding linen from the nurses.

100. You feel blessed every day because you have all your own teeth.

101. You are an under-appreciated reincarnation
of Mother Teresa!

About Neil Shulman, M.D....

Neil's comic personality has launched him into a successful career in entertainment where he has been using humor as therapy in a unique one-man traveling comedy show. Favorable reviews and publicity – from CNN, *U.S.A Today*, *The Miami Herald* – keep him booked before many audiences, from comedy clubs and colleges to national conferences to a United Nations peace mission in Cyprus. He philosophizes, performs monologues and tells of comic adventure, mixing the worlds of medicine, movies, and novels.

Shulman wrote the book *Doc Hollywood*, then co-produced the Michael J. Fox-starring motion picture his book inspired. Shulman's other fiction includes *The Backyard Tribe, Finally...I'm a Doctor, Life Before Sex, What's in a Doctor's Bag?, Under the Backyard Sky,* and *Second Wind.*

For speaking engagements, Shulman may be reached at (404) 321-0126, 2272 Vistamont Drive, Decatur, GA, 30033, nshulman@emory.edu or www.dochollywood.com

When you want to make a C.N.A. laugh…
Give a copy of *101 Ways to Know if You're a C.N.A.!!*

ORDER FORM (2 Pages)

Send checks to: Rx Humor
                  2272 Vistamont Dr., Decatur, GA 30033

or order via credit card at: www.dochollywood.com

Contact information: nshulma@bellsouth.net
                       Tel. (404) 321-0126 / fax (404) 633-9198

Mr./Mrs. _____

Address _____

City _____   State _____   Zip _____

Phone _____

☐ I have filled out the following page and included it with this page.
☐ I have enclosed a check or money order.

ORDER FORM

101 Ways to If Know You're a C.N.A.!!

    Quantity Ordered: _____

    Price per book (see below*): _____ *

    Cost: 1-9 copies = $9.00 each
              10-99 copies = $6.00 each
              100-999 copies = $4.00 each
              1000 or more = $3.00 each

    Subtotal: _____

    Shipping and handling ($1.00 for each book ordered): _____

    Sales Tax – 7% (GA Residents only): _____

    TOTAL AMOUNT DUE: _____